AF893723

Delilah

Delilah

The Journey

H. Etta

H. Etta

First Printing, 2020

Delilah

Delilah eats the cereal dry because the milk upsets her tummy.

She crunches down on it and swallows with a sip of black tea.

"Fit for a king," she says.

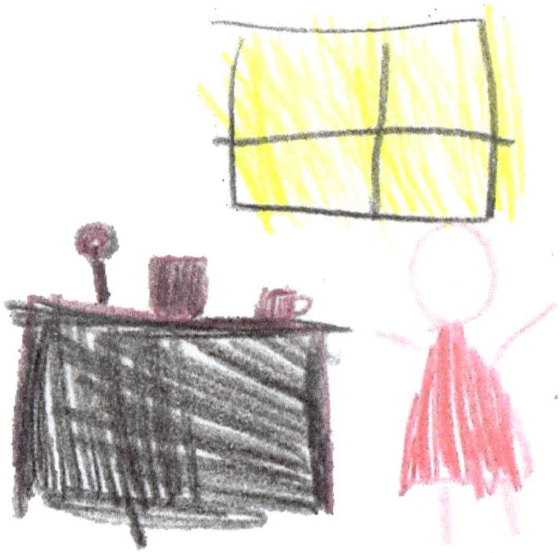

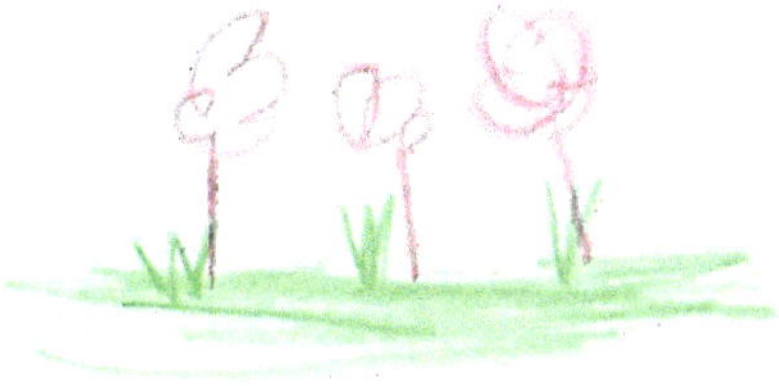

There is a bird with a broken wing in our garden.
It lives in a cardboard box now.
Rueben. Rueben likes to sing.

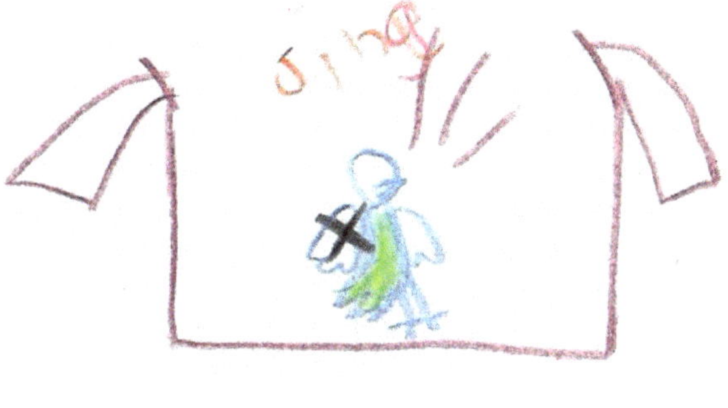

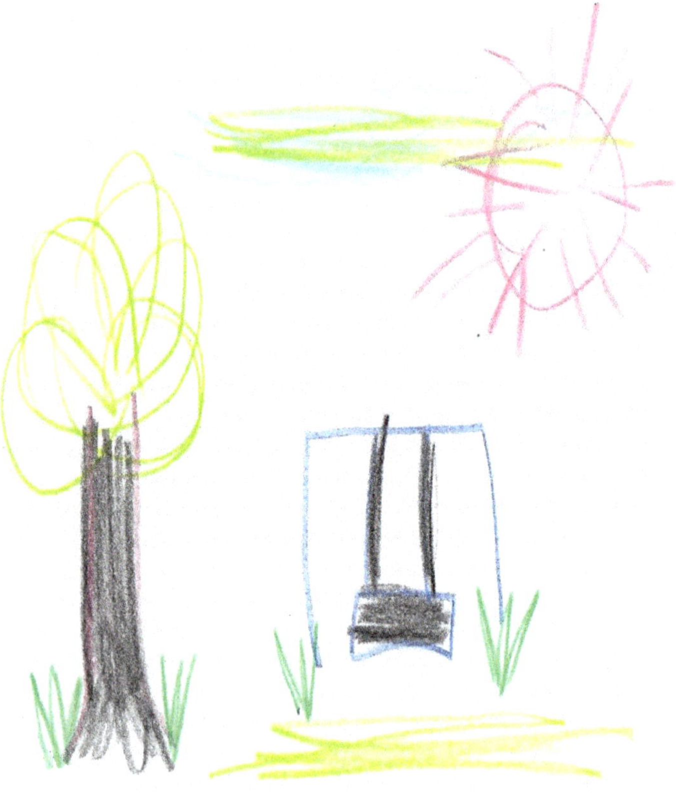

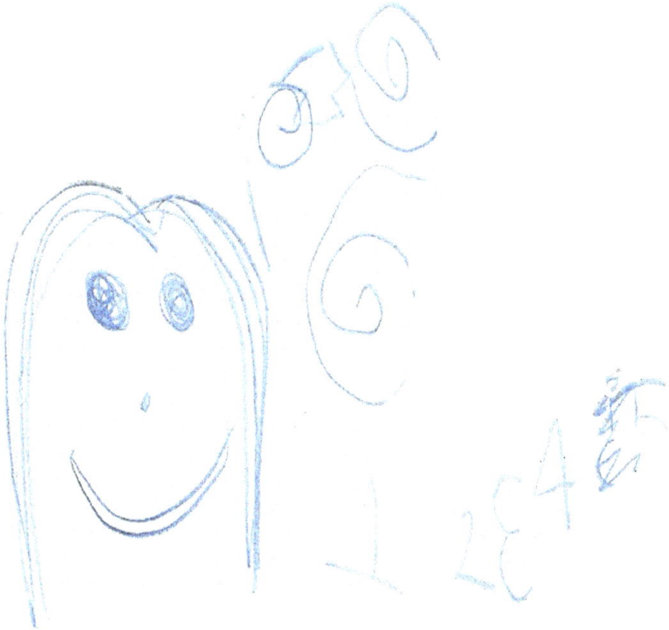

We take steps on the pavement and trip on our laces.
We laugh with our crooked teeth and we feel happy.

There's a journal on the bench that has reminders in it.

Thursday, we take Bumble for a walk. Friday, we have check-ups scheduled at two.

The check-ups only last ten minutes but we learn a lot.

More than we want to.

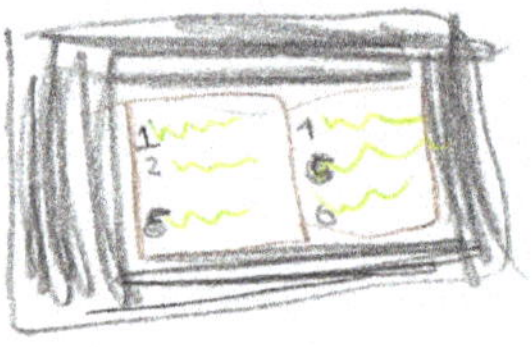

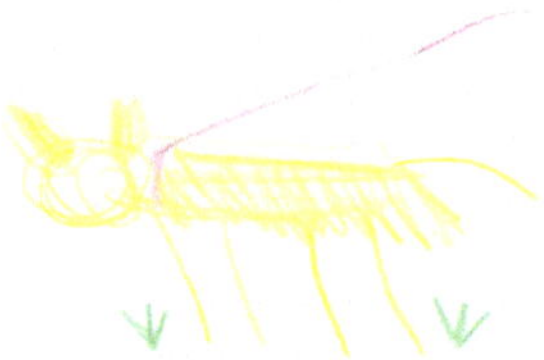

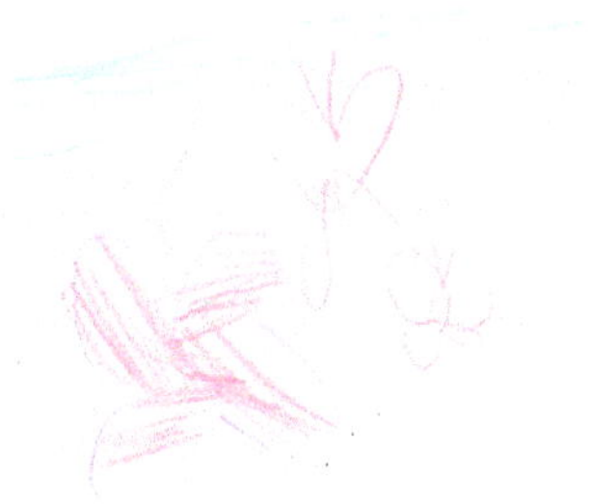

Bumble chases the butterflies and we can't keep up.

It's Friday.

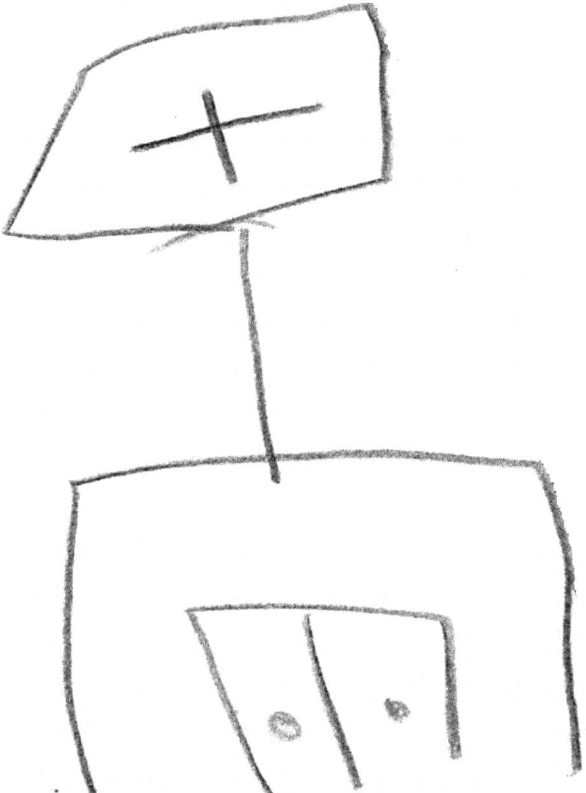

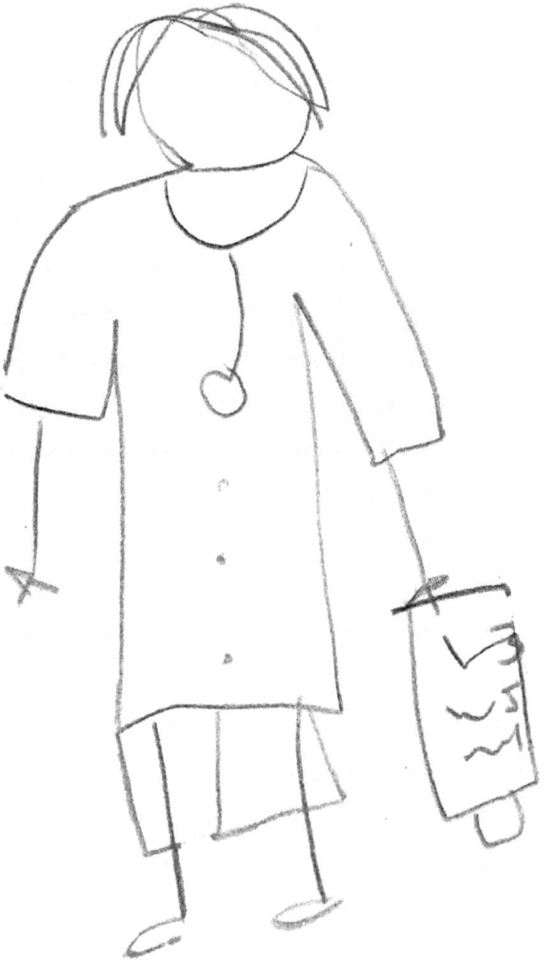

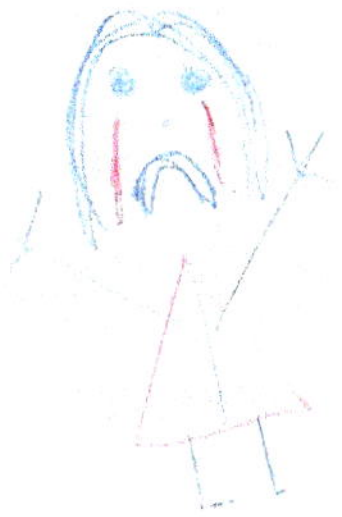

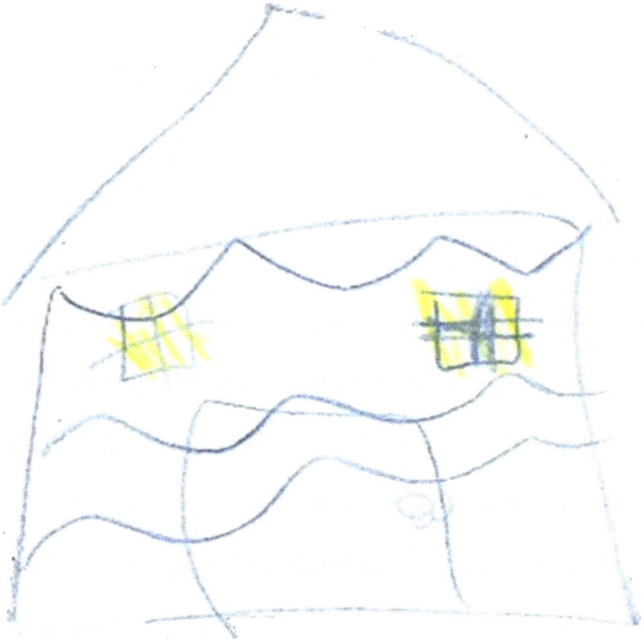

There's a hole in the wall and the drainpipes are leaking.

Delilah says there's no point fixing it.

Let the house flood.

I get scared.
Rueben is nestled in the box, not singing.
The floor is wet and my feet are cold.
Delilah is just smiling.

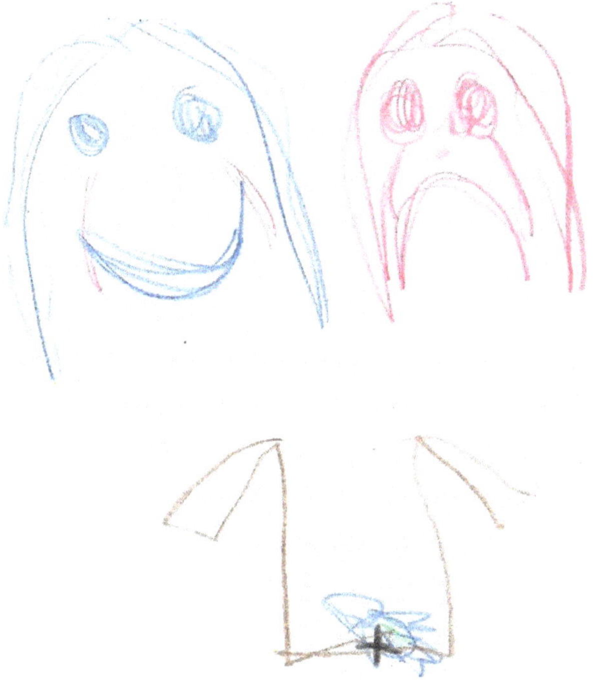

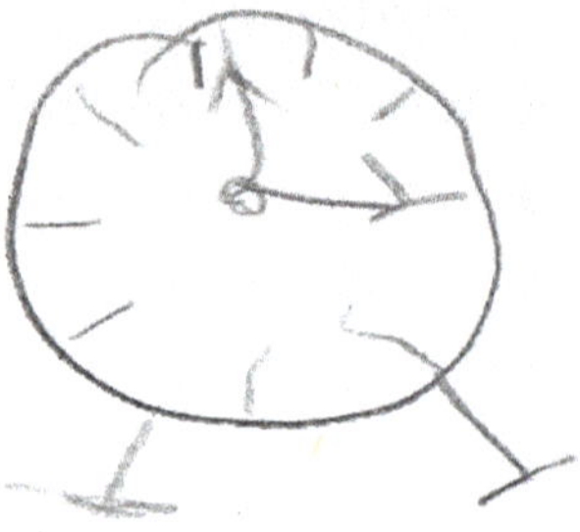

I crack my knuckles and place my bets.
A game of time and chance.
There is no birdsong to lull away the ache.
Goodbye Rueben.

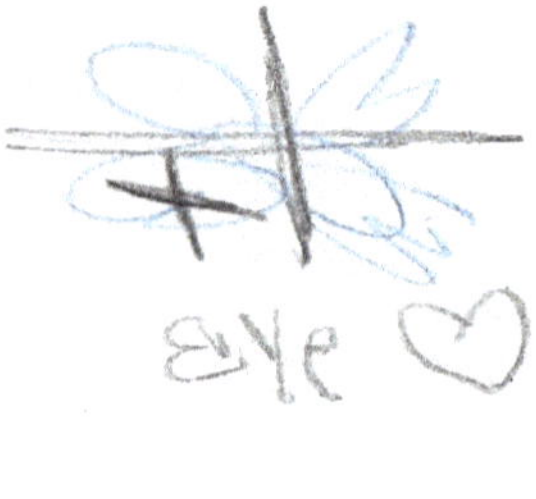

We put coloured stones on the dirt patch and we almost forget we are drowning.

Time to sit down.

More dry cereal.

Lots of coughing.

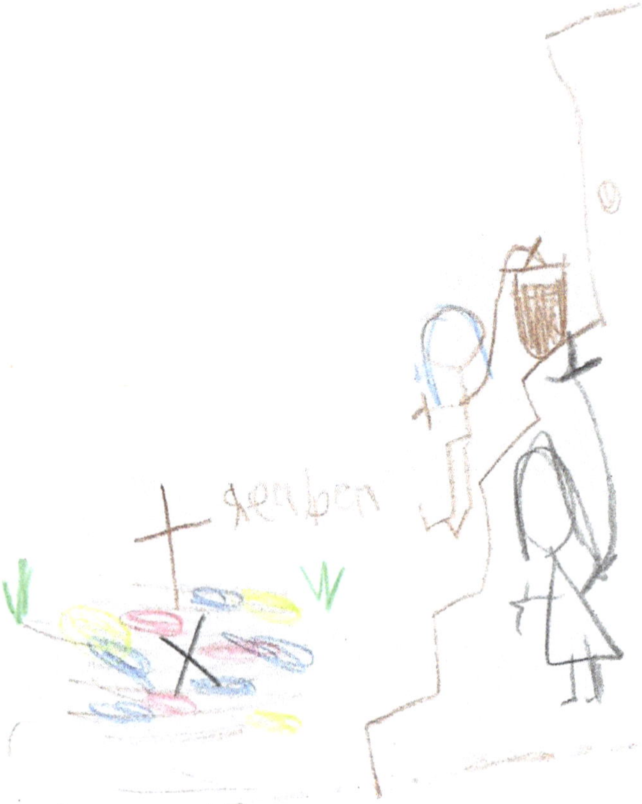

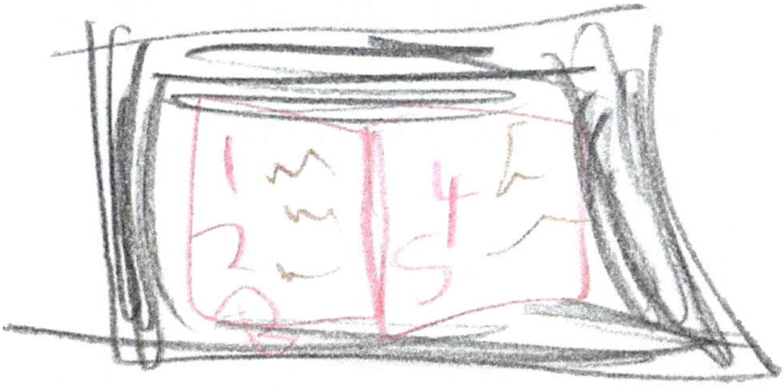

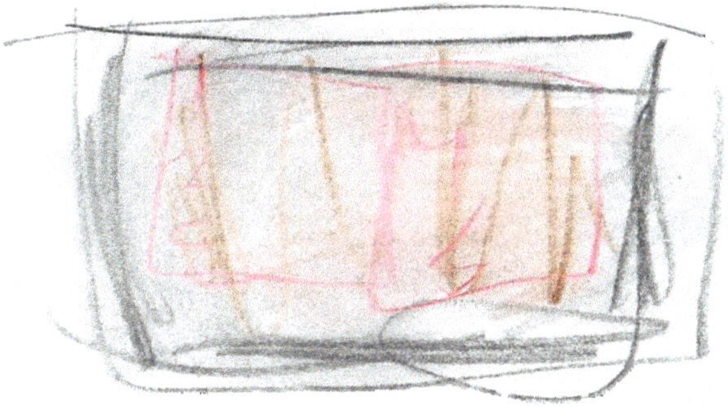

Tuesday is another check-up day.
The ink in the journal is smudged.
I can't read Wednesday.
I can't read Thursday.

Friday, we sit on the steps and tell Bumble sorry for not taking him for a walk on Thursday.

He sits in the sun unbothered.

We sit in the sun shivering.

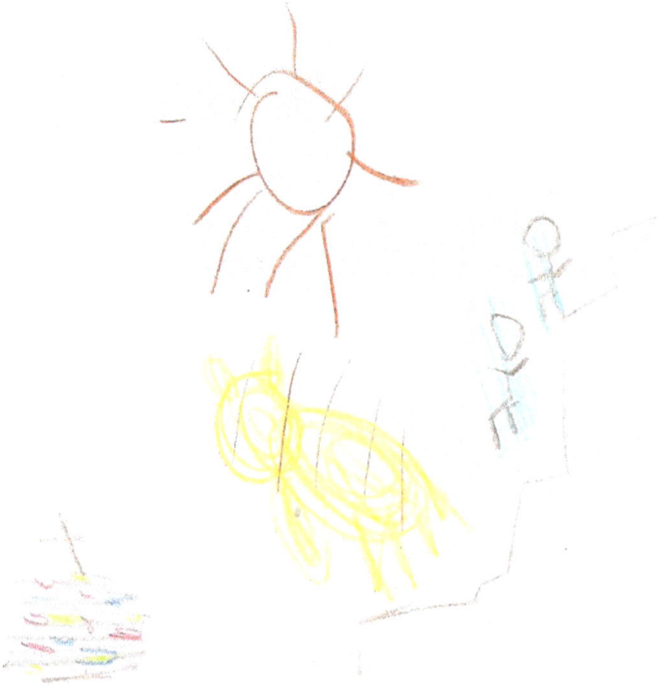

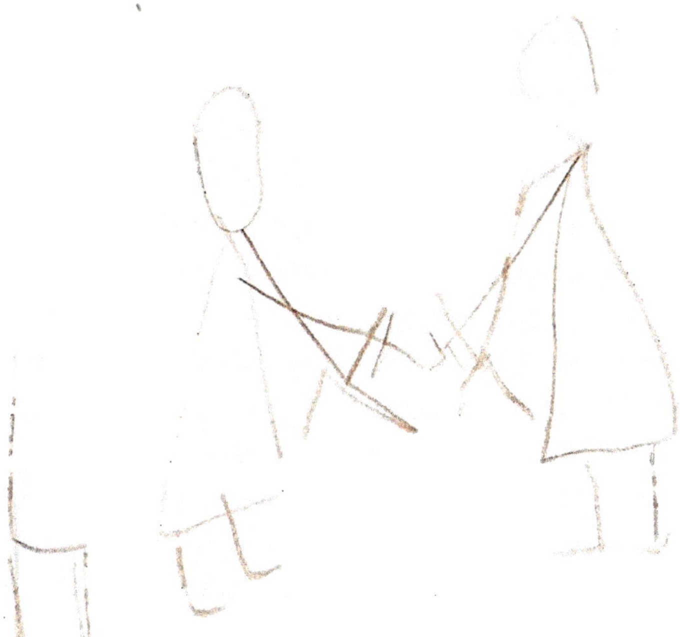

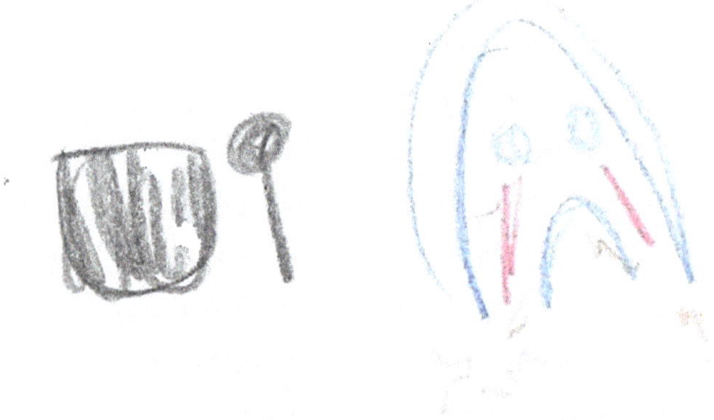

Delilah eats a full meal and splutters the whole time.

She says, "this is nice," while she chokes.

No more food after that, it is too easy to swallow wrong and she already can't breathe.

Today we got a phone call.
Tomorrow we get a new bed to sleep in.

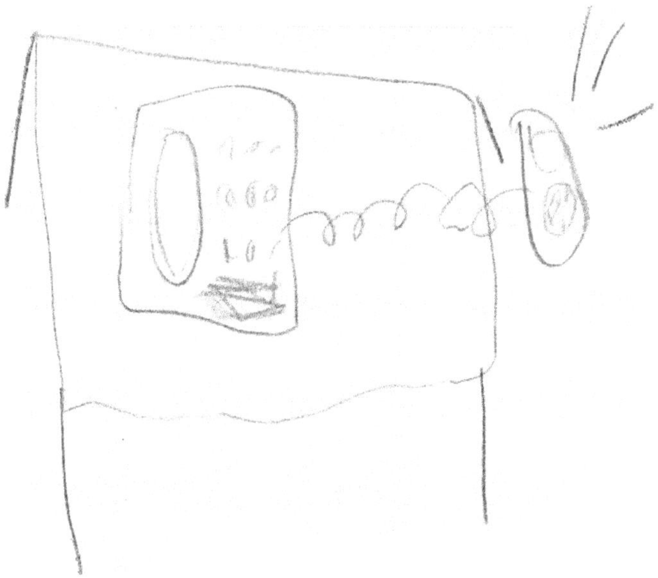

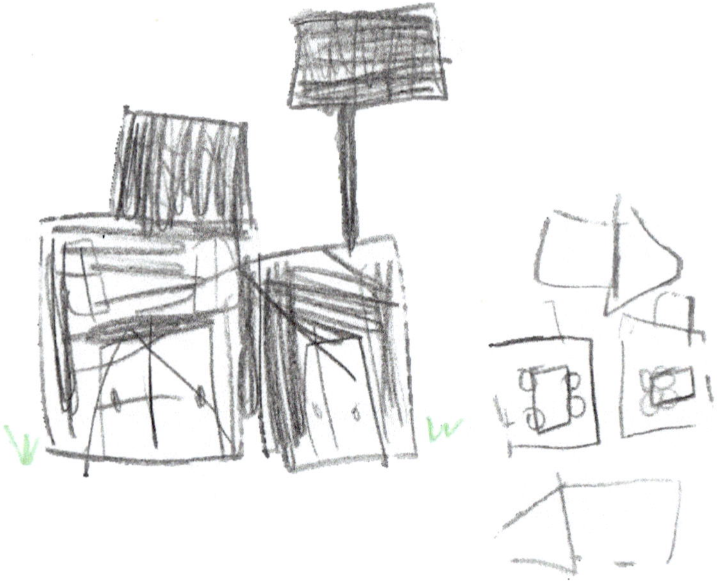

The sheets are stiff.
I am crying.
Delilah smiles and says thank you for the flowers.

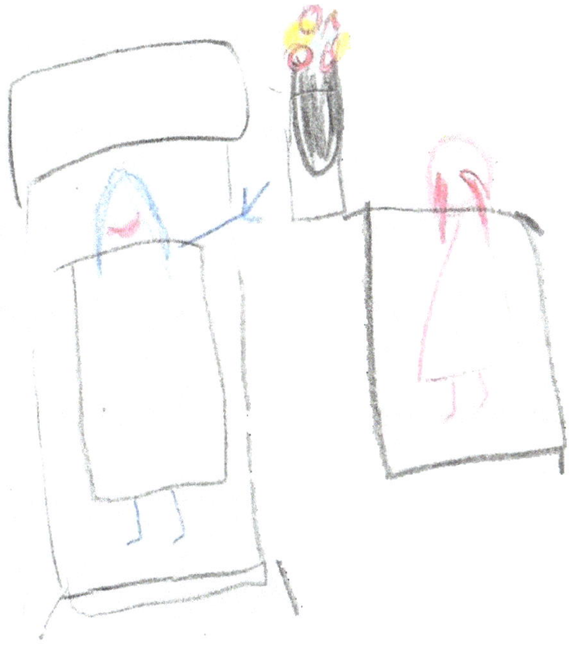

The windows are open of a morning.

There are 3 Ruebens that sing and Delilah sings too.

Delilah sings loud and unashamedly and the room lights up.

Delilah sings.

And that's the point.

I can hear her sing.

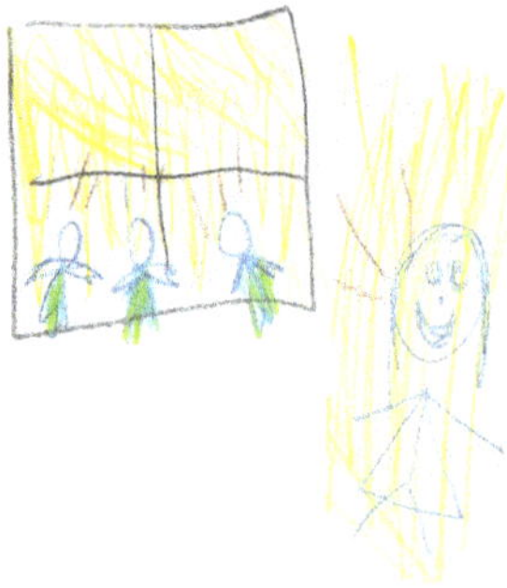

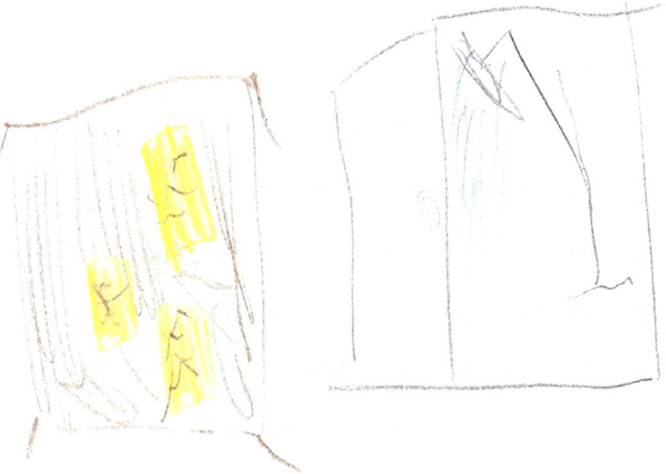

We write letters to Bumble.

Bumble can't read but it keeps us busy.

We shower five times.

Twice to clean the sick and an extra three times for warmth.

It is no home but it is where Delilah is safe.

We stay for so long.

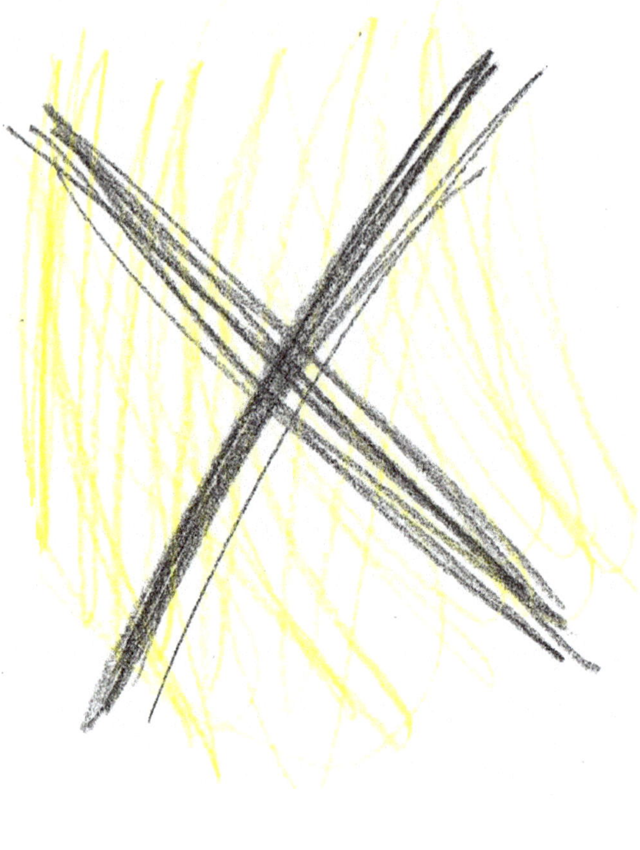

We tried to write stories today but adjectives are hard.
There's a word for this and I can only think of Delilah.
Delilah hurts.
I was going to keep quiet but I can't.

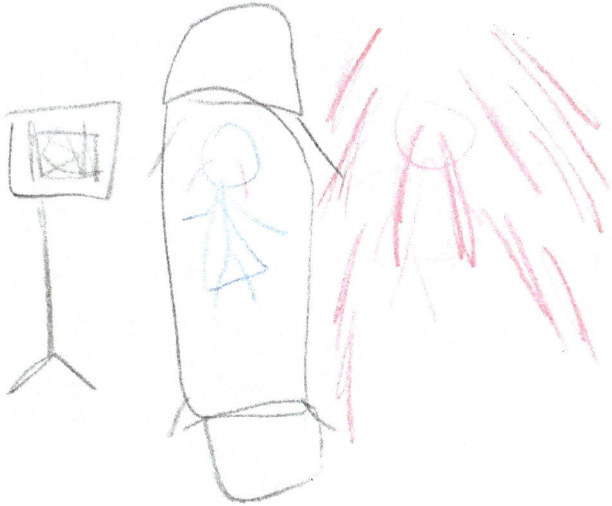

Only way to treat Delilah:
Morphine

Things that morphine cannot fix:
Delilah

Delilah:
Wakes up screaming so often now

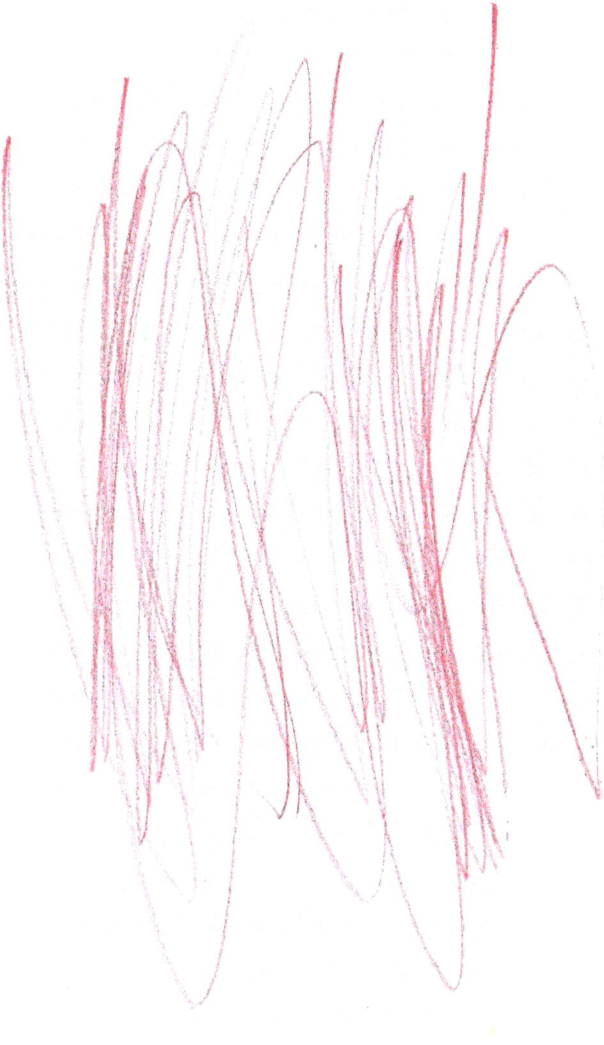

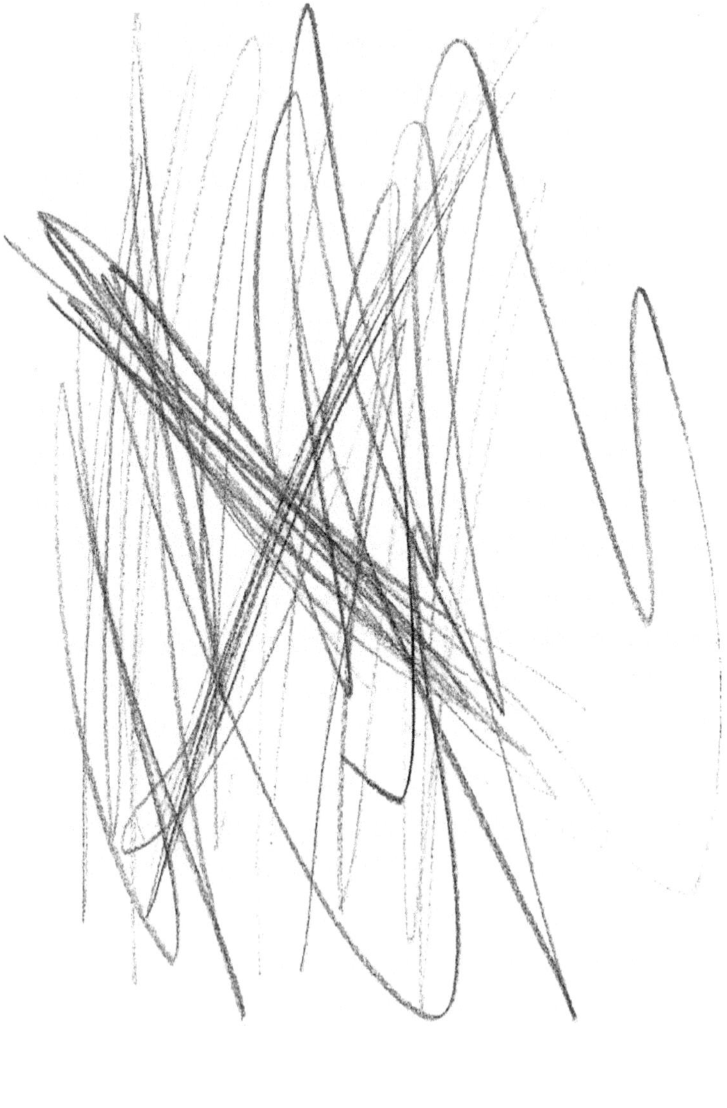

I am still here but The Sick killed us both.

H. Etta grew up in rural Australia and is fascinated by the array of notions, cultures and lifestyles that surround her. She is set on creating work that encapsulates the differing perspectives of those that she has never met from all of the places that she has never been. In short, she is a fiction writer; everything is manufactured using the imagination that only a small-town gal can have. H. Etta enjoys short walks to the nearby servo and decorates every meal with (entirely too much) Sriracha sauce. She hopes her work made you feel something - or anything at all and thanks you for your support in reading.

CPSIA information can be obtained
at www.ICGtesting.com
Printed in the USA
BVHW020351141020
590995BV00011BA/79

9 780646 827087